BY ANN DUGAN AND THE EDITORS OF
CONSUMER GUIDE®

NEW **7 DAY** PROGRAM

SLIMMING
YOUR
HIPS & THIGHS

Louis Weber, President
Publications International, Ltd.
3841 West Oakton Street
Skokie, Illinois 60076

Manufactured in the United States of America
10 9 8 7 6 5 4 3 2 1

Library of Congress Catalog Card Number: 83-60518
ISBN: 0-517-40838-4

Photography: Sam Griffith Studios, Inc.
Cover Design: Frank E. Peiler
Book Design: Ingeborg Jakobson

Contents

The 7 Day Program

*L*ooking sleek, trim, and healthy—
that's your goal. Slim hips and
thighs are essential to that lean look. Yet the
most common figure complaints are in that
area from the waist to the knees. These figure
problems are usually caused not only by excess
fat. They are caused also by muscles that are
out of shape. The muscles in this part of the
body are important in several ways. They
affect your energy level and your posture, as
well as your figure. When these muscles are
out of shape, you suffer threefold.

The New 7 Day Program for Slimming Your
Hips and Thighs is specifically designed to
firm up those muscles. No matter what shape
you're in now, you can look and feel better—
much sooner than you think.

You may have tried to diet off your extra
inches. Paying attention to what you eat is, of
course, essential to your health, fitness, and
figure. But weight loss alone will not give you
the firm, shapely figure you want. You need
well-toned muscles to have a good figure.
That's why you need a regular, carefully
planned exercise program.

The Slimming Your Hips and Thighs program gives you an exercise plan for every day
of the week. Each exercise routine takes only
about 30 minutes. The exercises are foolproof
and easy to follow. The entire program has
been designed to produce balanced muscle
development and shaping, while avoiding
injury and soreness. Follow this simple program, exercising regularly and vigorously each

day. You'll feel slimmer, firmer, stronger—
not just in your hips and thighs, but all over
your body.

If you really want the figure you've always
dreamed of, get this book out every day. Put
on some fast-paced music to swing you along.
You'll soon notice that you're looking a little
better every day you exercise. It will take
some effort, but it will all be worth it. Don't
expect overnight results. But within only a few
weeks, this program can change your figure
dramatically. It can shape you up enough to
make people say, "Gee, you look great."

Following the program

*T*he new Slimming Your Hips and
Thighs program offers 7 new exer-
cise routines—a different routine for every day
of the week. During the first 6 days, the program alternates days of lighter exercise with
days of more vigorous exercise, as recommended by medical experts on physical fitness.
At the same time, the exercises gradually pro-
gress from Day 1 on, so that Day 6 is the most
vigorous—and most beneficial—routine of the
week. Day 7 is a maintenance-level routine.
You might want to arrange your weekly exercise program so that you do the Day 7 routine
when you may have less time or energy to
devote to exercise, perhaps on the weekend.

Each of the 7 new routines includes warm-
up exercises, spot exercises for the hips and
thighs, stretches for flexibility, and cool-down

exercises. Most fitness experts agree that each type of exercise serves an important purpose. Each is essential to a sound fitness program.

Warm ups get your body going. They generally loosen up the muscles all over your body and get your heart and lungs working at higher levels. Warm ups are essential for two main reasons.

When your body is properly warmed up, the more vigorous hip and thigh exercises are more effective. Warm ups raise the body and muscle temperature to efficient levels. They increase the blood supply in the muscles and increase the rate and force of muscle contractions. Your car works more efficiently after the engine is warmed up. The same is true for your body.

Warm ups also make you less prone to injury when you go on to more vigorous exercises. They stretch the ligaments and tissues to permit greater flexibility. By gradually activating muscle fibers, you'll help prevent muscle tears and sprains. How will you know when you've warmed up enough? You'll be slightly out of breath, and you'll break the sweat barrier.

The exercises for the hips and thighs are a combination of spot exercises and stretches. Our *spot exercises* are muscle-toners, not "spot reducers." Exercising one area of the body will not reduce the amount of fat in that area. However, our spot exercises can change the shape of an area. Restoring muscle tone makes the hips and thighs firmer and more attractively shaped.

Stretches are often included as the last step in an exercise. Stretches help avoid injury by increasing flexibility and range of movement. The connective tissues of your body are like rubber bands. If not stretched frequently, the tissues become tight and limit your movement. If not stretched at all for a long time, the tissues may snap, causing injury and pain. Take the stretches slowly at first. Do not stretch any farther than you feel comfortable. As the ligaments gradually loosen, your stretches will go farther.

The hip and thigh exercises are carefully designed to help your muscles develop evenly. This even development of all the hip and thigh muscles is what gives you the shape and proportion you're after. Our exercise routines carefully alternate the muscles exercised. One exercise may work on the front of the leg; the next, on the back of the leg. One may work on the inside of the thigh; the next, on the outside. That is one more reason to do all the exercises in each routine in the order given.

Cool downs are exercises that allow your body to slow down gradually. After strenuous work, the body must readjust to pre-exercise levels of body function. Cool downs help your muscles begin to relax. They allow your circulatory system to slow down gradually. If you stop exercising suddenly, without this tapering-off period, blood collects in the muscles and veins. This could cause dizziness and weakness. A proper cool down also helps minimize stiffness and soreness.

Making it work

To get the most from the time and energy you put into this program, keep these guidelines in mind.

• Wear comfortable clothing that allows you to move freely, such as shorts, a leotard, or a light exercise suit.

• Exercise in tennis shoes, in socks, or barefoot—whatever is most comfortable to you. If you have a weak back, weak knees, or weak ankles, wear tennis shoes or running shoes. You may sometimes need to remove shoes, however, for exercises that require sliding the feet on the floor.

• If possible, exercise on a wooden floor or on a carpet. Exercising on concrete surfaces can be hard on your body. For floor exercises, try to work on a mat, a carpet remnant, a piece of foam rubber, or a folded towel.

• When doing chair exercises, use a sturdy chair with a firm base. Be sure the chair is strong enough to support your weight. As an extra caution, place the chair under a table to prevent its tipping over. You may also lean on a windowsill or a kitchen counter, instead of a chair, for these exercises.

• Try to exercise every day, or at least four times a week. A regular exercise program offers the most benefit for your body.

• Establish your own exercise schedule. You shouldn't exercise just before bedtime or just after you eat. Most any other time is fine. Once you choose the best time, stick to it. Exercising at the same time every day helps you develop the exercise habit.

• Follow the routines carefully. If you follow directions, you should tone and shape muscles properly, avoid injury, and suffer a minimum of soreness.

• If you cannot do an exercise exactly as it is described, don't worry. Try it, and then go on to the next exercise. Don't feel discouraged. As you increase your strength and flexibility, you will eventually be able to do most of the exercises. Then you will realize just how far you have progressed.

• Remember that your individual body structure may make an exercise difficult for you. Body structure and flexibility vary greatly from person to person. The structure of your joints or the length of your arms or legs may prevent you from doing an exercise exactly as it is described. Don't push yourself past your own body's limits. Aim toward what is asked for in each exercise, doing the best that you can.

• Do the number of repetitions given in the text, until the exercises are easy for you. Then gradually increase the number of repetitions for each exercise. For some exercises, the text recommends the number of repetitions you should try to work toward. In general, you might aim toward eventually doubling the repetitions given in the text. But don't try to go too far too fast. Don't try to double the repetitions all at once. Add only 3 to 5 repetitions at a time, until that number becomes easy.

• At the end of each day's exercises, you should feel a healthy, relaxed sense of fatigue. Exercise that does not tax the body does not help the body.

• No matter how rushed you may be, do not neglect to do the warm ups and cool downs. These exercises are essential for keeping your body flexible, getting your heart and lungs working efficiently, and avoiding injury and stiffness.

• As you work through each day's routine, keep your body moving. You lose some of the benefits if you take long breaks between exercises. Exercising to lively music can help you pace yourself and really keep you going.

• Learn to listen to your own body for signs of fatigue. You want to exercise vigorously enough to work up a sweat. But be careful not to overdo. If you're winded and breathless, or if you suffer sprains or stitches in the side, assume that you're exercising too vigorously. Slow down a little.

• If you haven't exercised for a while, it is normal to be a little sore and stiff when you first start. Stiffness does not mean you should stop moving. In most cases, it means you should get going again. Remember that warming up and cooling down properly will help minimize soreness.

• If you think you may be injured, stop using the injured limb. Continuing to exercise could worsen the injury. Stop your exercise program until the injury no longer hurts when you are at rest. Then gradually begin to exercise slowly and carefully.

• If you have a weak back, weak ankles, or weak knees, be careful during exercises that put stress on those parts of the body. Those exercises will eventually strengthen the muscles in those areas. But go slowly until you build up that strength.

• Supplement this program with as much activity as possible. You should consciously aim at becoming a more physically active person. Try to do more walking, bicycling, dancing. Take the stairs instead of the elevator. Participate in whatever active sports you enjoy. Keep that energy level up.

• Don't be discouraged if you gain a little weight after the first week of exercise. A small weight gain means that the muscles are becoming firmer and denser. Those few extra pounds will disappear after another week of regular exercise.

• If you miss a week or more on this program, start again with the number of repetitions given in the text. You'll have to rebuild your strength and flexibility before increasing the number of repetitions again.

• All the exercises in this program were developed in consultation with medical experts. However, it is recommended that you consult your doctor before beginning this or any program of exercise.

Let's get going

Now you're ready to begin. You have the ground rules. You understand how this terrific program works. So get into some comfortable clothes, put some upbeat music on the stereo, and let's get moving. Remember, the hips and thighs are quick to respond to a well-designed exercise program. You could feel better and start looking firmer and slimmer by next week!

DAY 1

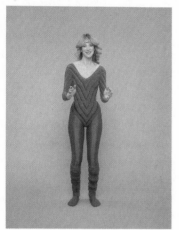

Starting position

Warm up
Reach and run

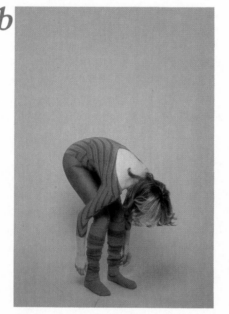

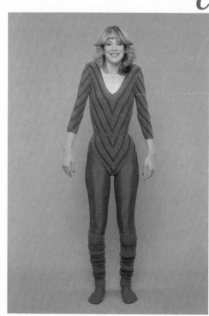

Assume starting position.

a Slowly run in place, lifting the knees and landing lightly on the feet. While running, reach one arm then the other straight upward. Alternate arms with each step. Reach and run for 40 counts.

b Bend the knees and round the back over until hands dangle at the ankles. Hold 5 counts. To return to upright position, slowly press the hips forward, straighten the legs, uncurl the back, and raise the head.

c Raise the shoulders as high as possible. Hold 5 counts. Lower. Raise and lower shoulders twice.

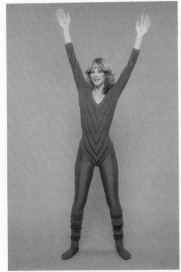

Starting position

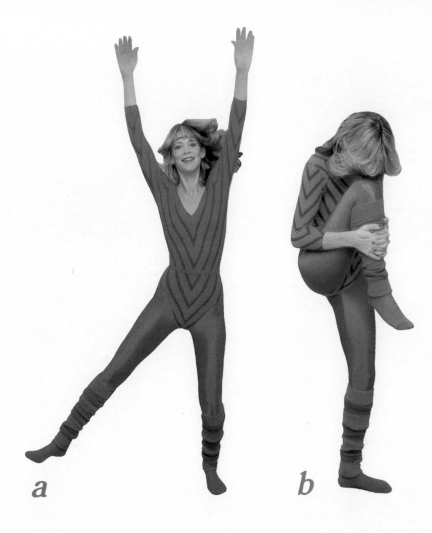

a

b

Warm up
Swing and circle

Assume starting position

a Kick right leg out to the side and return to center. Landing on right foot, kick left leg out to the side and return. While kicking side to side, circle arms up overhead, around, down, and up again. Kick side to side 20 times.

b Pull knee to chest. Hold for 5 counts, while slowly pressing the nose to the knee. Lower leg to floor. Repeat 3 times with each leg.

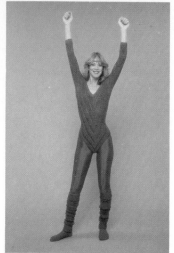

Starting position

Super swing

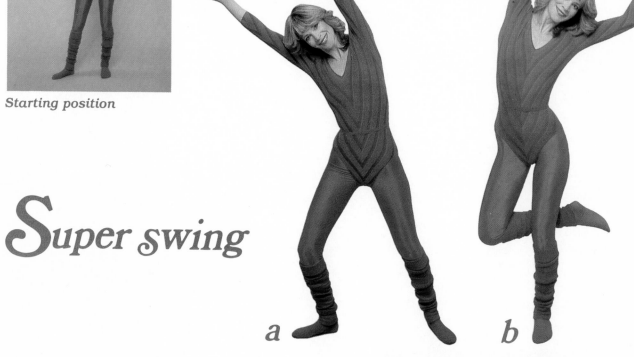

a

b

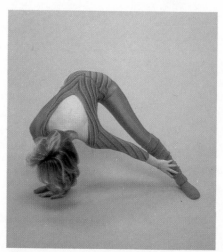

c

Assume starting position.

a Lunge to the right, leaning over bent right knee, swinging arms overhead to the right.

b Pushing off the right foot, cross right leg up behind the left leg. At the same time, swing arms down, across, and up to the left. Lunge and kick up 4 times with each leg. Work up to 8 times each leg.

c Assume the lunge position with right knee bent. Place right hand on the floor by the right foot. Hold left ankle with the left hand. Slowly straighten the right leg as much as possible. Hold for 5 counts. Relax. Repeat 3 times to each side.

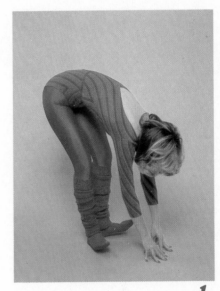
Starting position

Contour sit

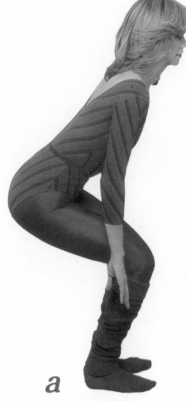
a

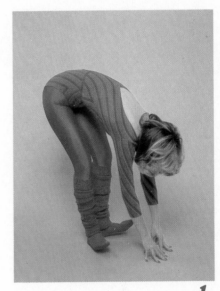
b

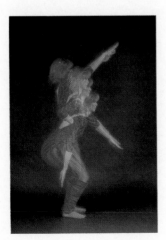

Assume starting position.

a Slowly bend knees, lowering the hips, keeping the back straight. Swing arms down toward the ankles. Continue swinging arms forward and up, straightening legs to return to an upright position. Repeat 10 times. Use the legs (not the back) to lower and raise the body.

b Bend knees and place fingertips on the floor in front of the feet. Lift toes. Pivoting on the heels, slowly turn toes out to the sides and in again. Repeat 8 times.

Knee press I

a Keeping the back straight, pull the knees in, swinging arms to the front. Return knees and arms to starting position. Repeat 8 times. Do not lower hips below the knees.

b Stand. Bend left leg back. Grasp ankle with the left hand. Pull the ankle up as far as possible. Do once with each leg.

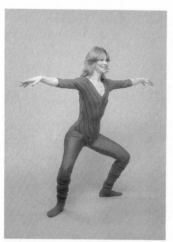

Starting position

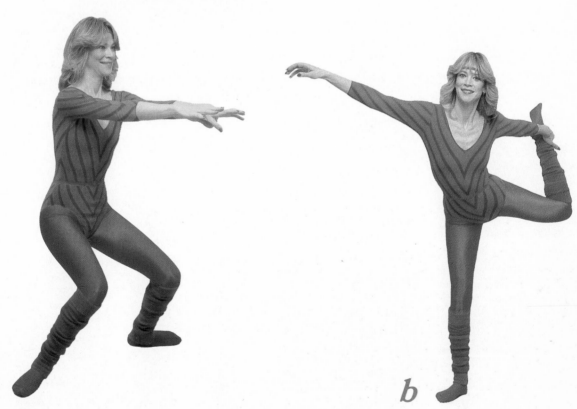

a

b

Thigh trimmer

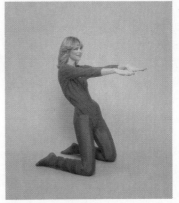

Starting position

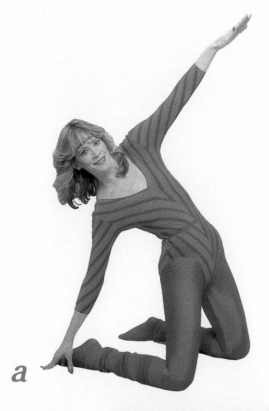

a

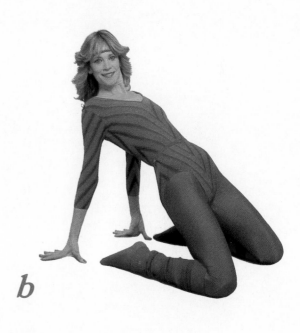

b

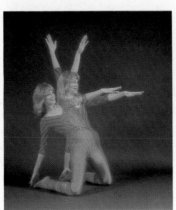

Assume starting position.

a Lean torso back. Touch the right hand to the floor by the right foot. Return to starting position. Repeat with the left hand. Touch right hand then left hand 4 times. Work up to 8 times.

b Keeping torso straight, lean back to place both hands on the floor. Hold and stretch for 3 counts. Push off the floor with both hands to return to starting position. Repeat 3 times.

Swing out

Assume starting position.

a Swing right leg forward, trying to touch the right elbow to the right knee. Return to starting position. Repeat 10 times with each leg.

b Rest for 5 counts. In starting position, bend the right knee. Grasp the foot with the right hand. Slowly try to straighten the leg. Then lift the leg as high as possible. Repeat 3 times with each leg.

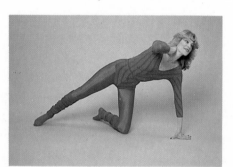

Starting position

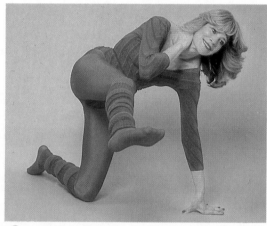

a

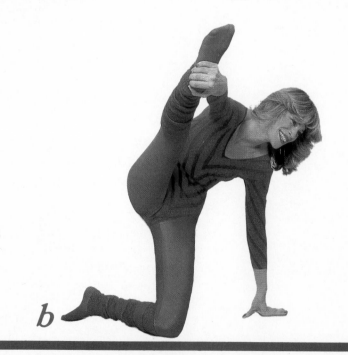

b

Cool down
Scissors stretch

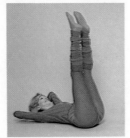

Starting position

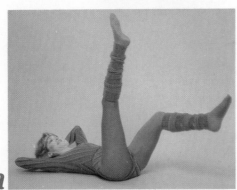

a

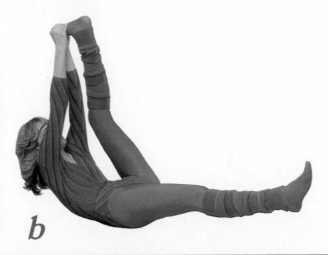

b

Assume starting position.

a Lower left leg toward the floor, while bringing right leg toward the head. Then reverse leg positions, bringing left leg toward the head, right leg toward the floor. Repeat 30 times.

b Grasp left foot with both hands. Slowly try to straighten the leg. Hold for 5 counts. Do once with each leg.

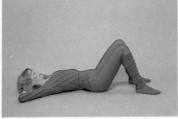

Starting position

Cool down
Hip hooray

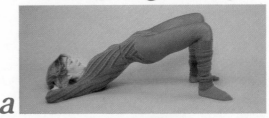

a

Assume starting position.

a Lift hips off the floor as high as possible. Hold for 5 counts.

b Keeping hips off the floor, lift the right leg toward the head as far as possible. Hold for 5 counts. Return leg to the floor. Do once with each leg.

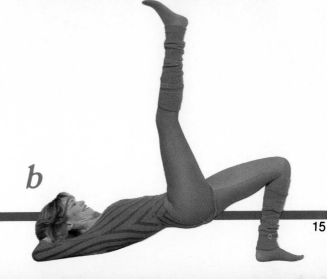

b

DAY 2

Assume starting position.

a Hop on left foot, touching right heel to floor. Twist torso to the right, keeping arms to the left.

b Hop on left foot again, touching right toe to the floor. Twist torso to the left, swinging arms to the right. Heel and toe, swinging arms back and forth, 20 times with each foot. Gradually work up to 35 times with each foot.

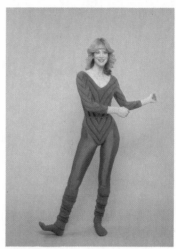

Starting position

Warm up
Heel-toe jig

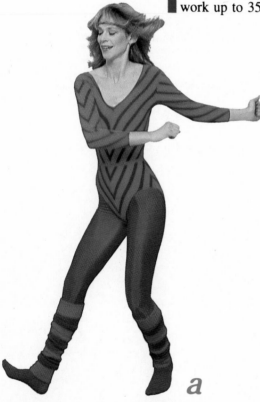

a

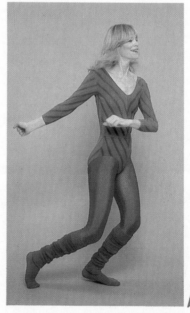

b

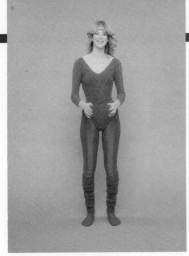

Starting position

Warm up
The cheerleader

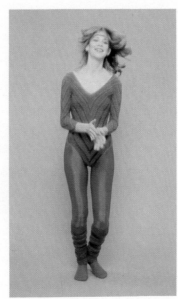

b

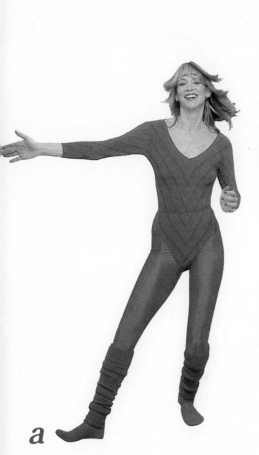

a

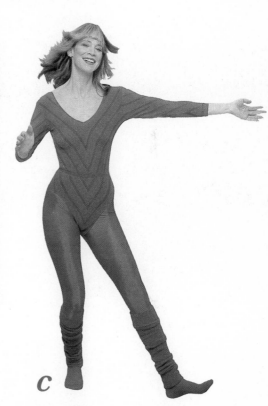

c

Assume starting position.

a Hop on left foot, touching right foot to floor out to the side. Swing right arm out to the side.

b Jump, feet together, and clap hands.

c Hop on right foot, touching left foot to floor out to the side. Swing left arm out to the side. Return to jump and clap. Repeat 16 times.

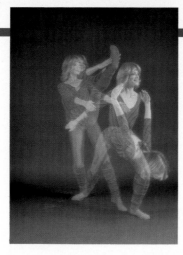

The kicker

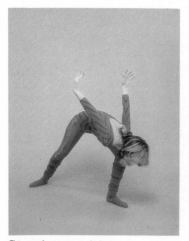

Starting position

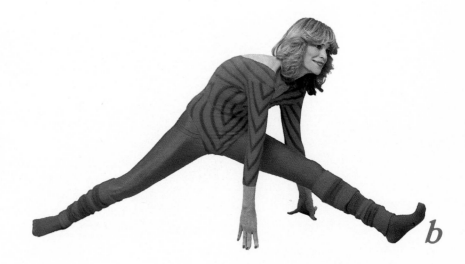

b

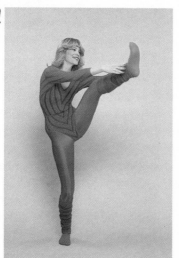

a

Assume starting position.

a Push off the left foot, shifting weight to the right leg. Kick the left leg as high as possible, touching hands to the ankle. Do 4 times with each leg. Repeat this sequence 3 times.

b In starting position, place hands on the floor, one on each side of the front leg. Very slowly slide the front leg forward as far as is comfortable. Do once with each leg.

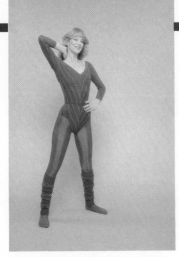

Starting position

Double dip

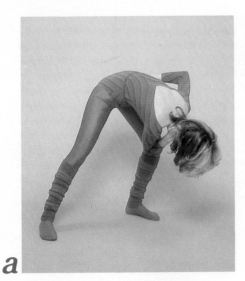

a

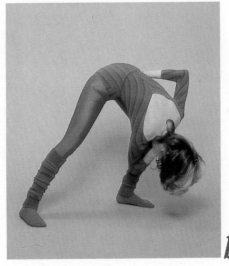

b

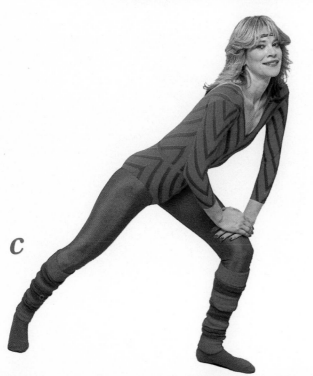

c

Assume starting position.

a Bending the left knee, bring right elbow down to the knee. Return to starting position.

b Bending knee again, bring elbow down to the calf. Return to starting position. Alternate bringing the elbow to the knee then to the calf. Repeat 8 times on each side.

c Bend left knee. Extend right leg straight back, toe on the floor. Place hands on left knee. Hold for 10 counts. Then lift and lower the hips 5 times. Repeat to the right side.

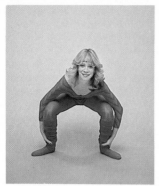
Starting position

Assume starting position.

a Holding outside of ankles, pull the knees in toward each other. Then press knees out. Repeat 8 times. Work up to 16 times. Do not lower hips below the knees.

b Place right hand on the floor. Bend right leg back. Grasp right foot with left hand. Pull the leg up and away from the body. Hold 5 counts. Do once with each leg.

Knee press II

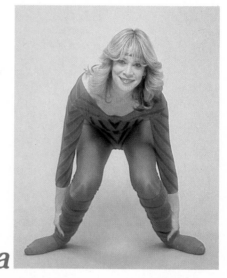
a

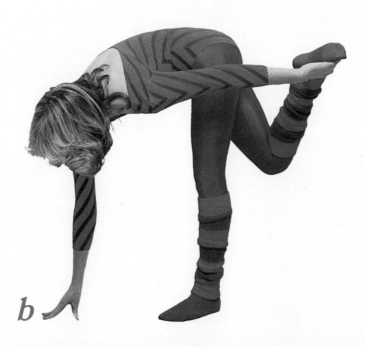
b

Assume starting position.

a Swinging arms out to sides, cross left leg behind the right. Left foot on the floor, both knees bent, slowly press the left knee down toward the right calf. Hold 5 counts. Return to starting position. Repeat 8 times with each leg.

b Do the same movement, but try to touch the knee to the floor. Turn the palms up. Hold 5 counts. Return to starting position. Repeat 5 times with each leg. If you have weak knees, do not touch knee to the floor or bend knee too low.

The curtsy

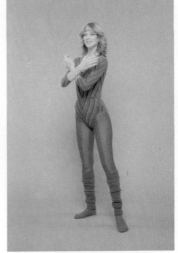

Starting position

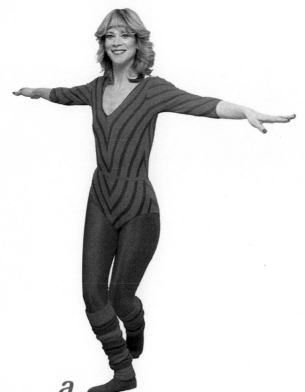

a

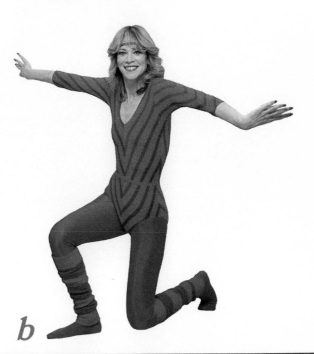

b

The tightener

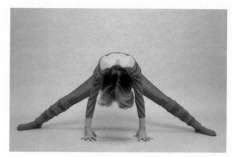

Starting position

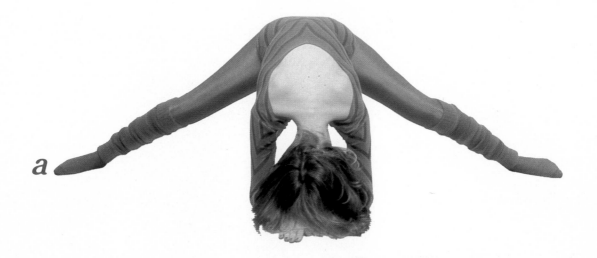

a

Assume starting position.

a Bend elbows down toward the floor. Then straighten the arms. Repeat 8 times. As you build strength, try to place elbows on the floor.

b Do the same exercise with the toes up, weight on the heels. Repeat 8 times.

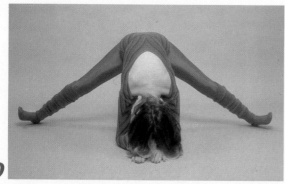

b

Cool down
Rag doll

a Bending knees, swing arms down between the legs, bending forward from the waist. Swing back up to starting position. Repeat 5 times.

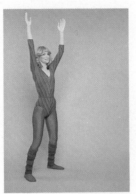

Starting position

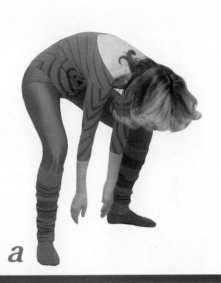

a

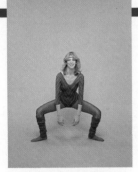

Starting position

Assume starting position.

a Swing arms up to the right, straightening legs and turning torso to the right. Stretch. Return to starting position. Repeat to the left side. Swing right then left 10 times.

Cool down
The swinger

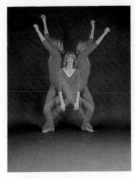

a

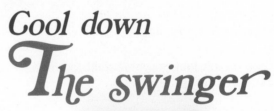

DAY 3

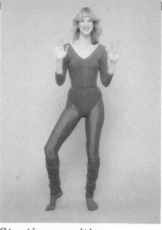

Starting position

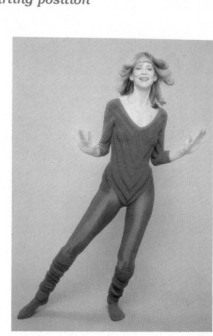

Warm up
Dixie shuffle I

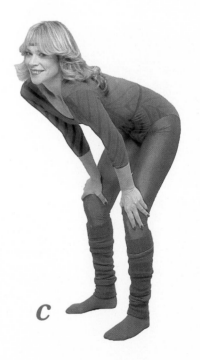

a

b

c

Assume starting position.

a Hop on left foot, touching right foot to the floor in front of the left foot.

b Hop on left foot again, touching right foot to the floor at the right side. While touching foot left and right, move hands in small circles. Touch left and right 15 times with each foot.

c Place hands on bent knees. Lift the shoulders. Hold for 5 counts. Lower shoulders. Repeat 3 times. Slowly uncurl the back to return to an upright position.

Warm up
Dixie shuffle II

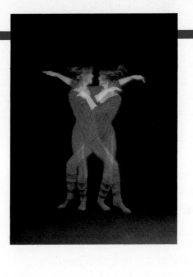

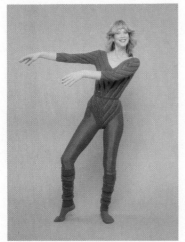

Starting position

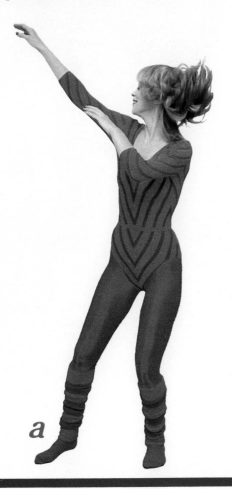

a

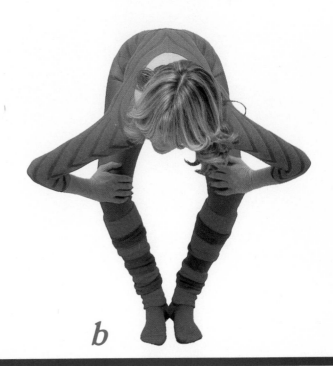

b

Assume starting position.

a Hop on left foot, touching right toe to floor at the right side. Turn torso to the right, arms right. Jump, feet together, swinging arms down. Then hop on right foot, touching left toe to the floor at the left side. Swing arms and torso to the left. Return to jump, arms down. Repeat 20 times.

b Stand with feet together, hands on bent knees. Press knees out to the sides. Hold 5 counts. Bring knees together. Repeat 3 times.

Assume starting position.

a Keeping heels on the floor, rock the knees side to side. Swing the arms side to side at the same time. Rock knees left and right 20 times.

b With right knee bent, extend the left leg with the toes up. Lowering hips, try to touch hands to the floor, one hand on each side of the left foot. Hold 5 counts. Repeat with right leg extended. Do once with each leg.

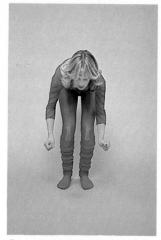

Starting position

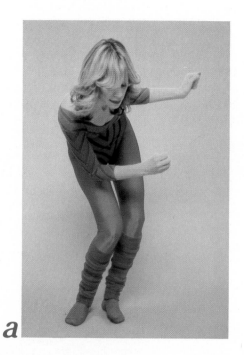

a

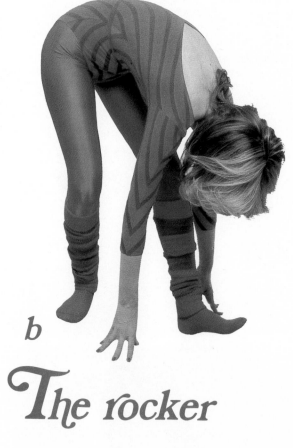

b

The rocker

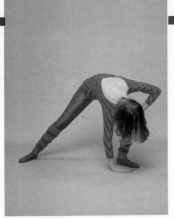

Starting position

The little dipper

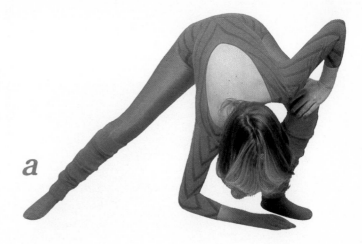

a

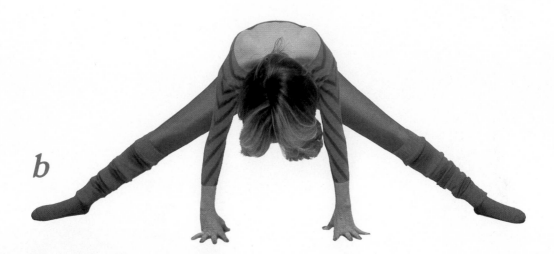

b

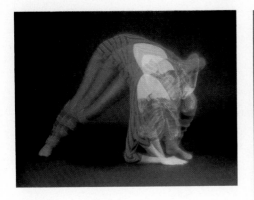

Assume starting position.

a Keep right hand on floor in front of left foot, left hand on knee to support the back. Bending left knee lower, bend the right elbow down toward the floor. Then straighten the elbow and straighten left leg as much as possible. Repeat 10 times to each side.

b Place feet wide apart, knees slightly bent. Put hands on the floor, head down. Slide feet out as wide as possible. Then pull feet in toward each other. Repeat 5 times. Remove shoes to slide feet more easily on the floor.

Knee lifter

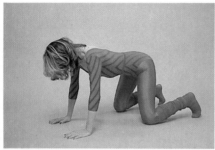

Starting position

Assume starting position.

a Lift knees off the floor about 12 inches. Then lower knees to about 2 inches off the floor. Repeat 10 times without returning knees to the floor.

b From starting position, lift knees off the floor. Straighten the legs as much as possible. Try to press the heels back toward the floor. Return to starting position. Repeat 10 times.

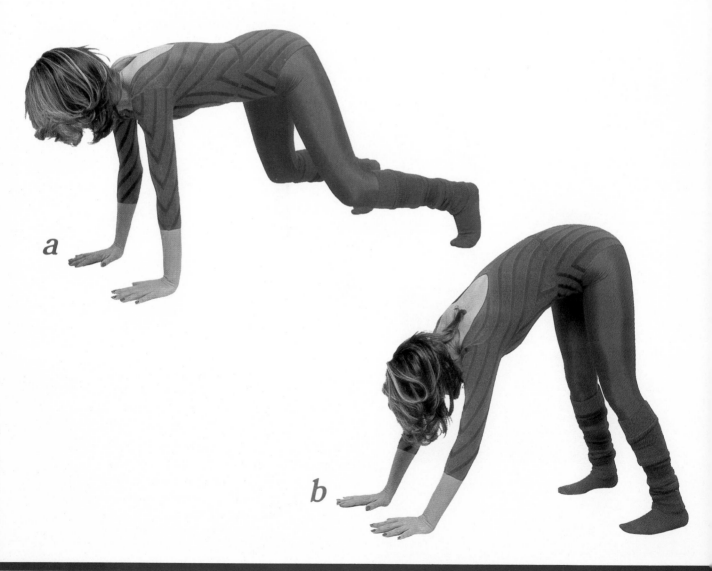

a

b

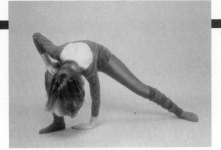

Starting position

The big dipper

Assume starting position.

a Keep left hand behind the right heel, right hand on knee to support the back. Bending right knee lower, bend the left elbow down toward the floor. Then straighten the elbow and straighten right leg as much as possible. Repeat 10 times to each side.

b Put hands on the floor, head down. Place feet wide apart, weight on the heels with the toes up. Slide heels out as wide as possible. Then pull heels in toward each other. Repeat 5 times. Remove shoes to slide feet more easily on the floor.

a

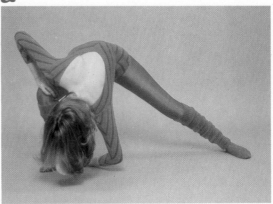

b

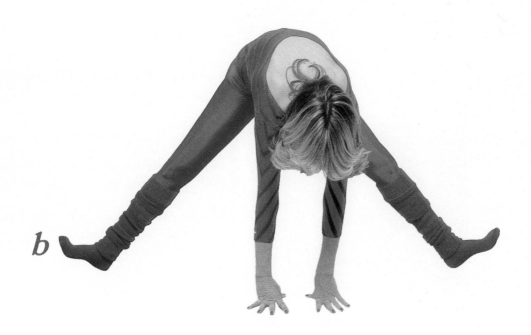

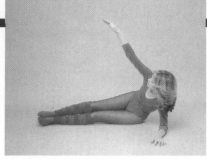

Starting position

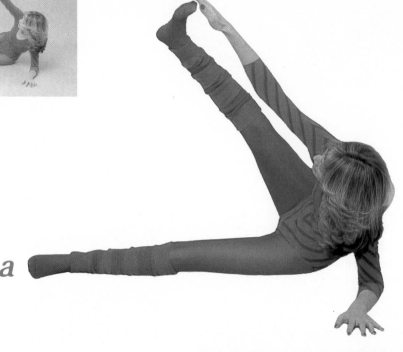

a

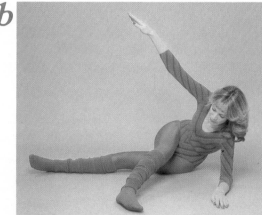

b

Cross kick

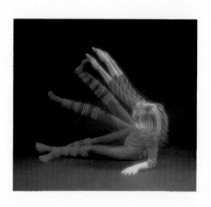

Assume starting position.

a Raise right leg up to the side as high as possible. Touch toes with the right hand.

b Lower the leg, crossing to touch the floor in front of the left leg. Return to starting position. Repeat 15 times with each leg.

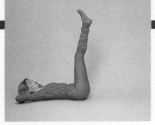

Starting position

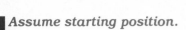

Cool down
Get your kicks

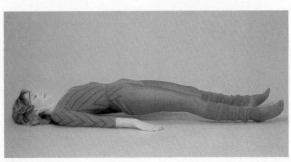

a

Assume starting position.

a Alternately kick right leg then left leg straight up for 5 counts. Alternately kick left leg then right leg forward for 5 counts. Repeat, kicking up then forward, 20 times.

b Lower legs to the floor. Place the hands at the sides, palms down. Lift the hips off the floor. Hold 5 counts. Lower hips. Repeat 3 times.

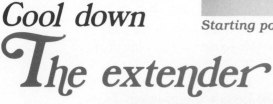

b

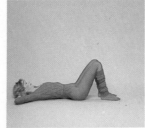

Starting position

Assume starting position.

a Lifting feet off the floor, bend knees in toward the chest. Then extend both legs straight up.

b Bend knees in toward the chest again. Then extend legs forward. Repeat the sequence (knees to chest, legs up, knees to chest, legs forward) 20 times.

Cool down
The extender

a

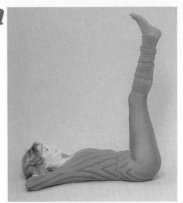

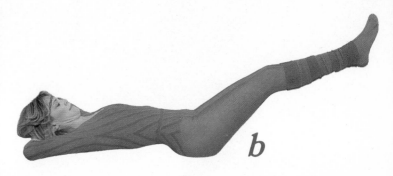

b

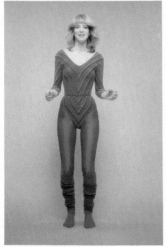

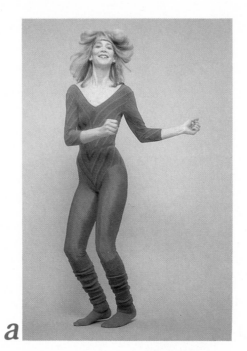

Starting position

a

Warm up
Do the twist

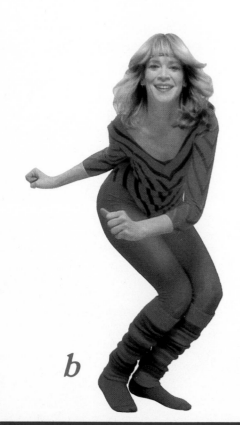

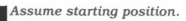

Assume starting position.

a With feet slightly apart, twist the body left then right, pivoting on the balls of the feet. Swing the arms side to side at the same time. Twist right and left 10 times.

b Now bend the knees and hips lower. Twist right and left 5 times. Repeat the sequence (twisting 10 times upright, 5 times bent low) 3 times.

b

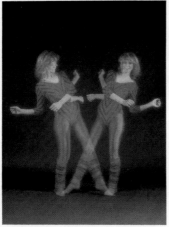

Warm up
Let's twist again

Assume starting position.

a Keep feet wide apart. Lean body to the left. Twist for 5 counts, pivoting on the balls of the feet. Swing the arms back and forth at the same time. Now lean to the right and twist for 5 counts. Repeat the sequence (twisting 5 counts leaning left, 5 counts leaning right) 3 times.

b Stand, weight on the left leg. Pull the right leg up, holding the foot with both hands. Press the foot away from the body. Hold for 5 counts. Do once with each leg.

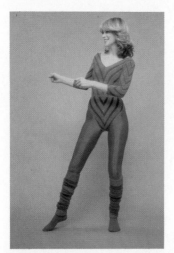

Starting position

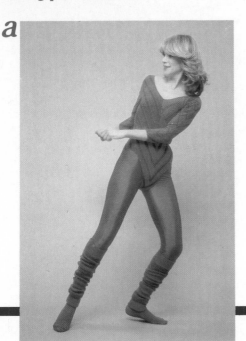

a

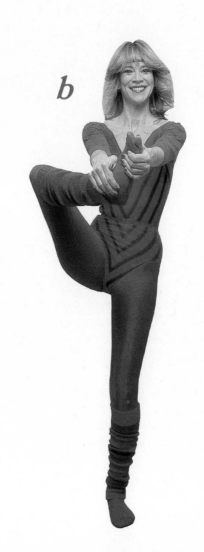

b

Knee pull-up

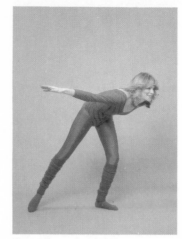

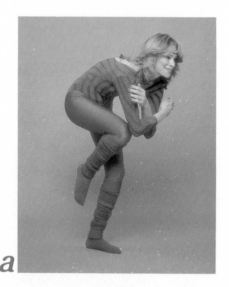

a

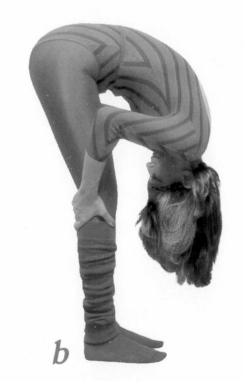

b

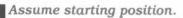

Assume starting position.

a Keep the left knee bent. Lift the right foot off the floor, bringing the knee up toward the chest. At the same time, cross the arms in front of the chest. Return to starting position. Repeat 10 times with each leg.

b Stand with feet together, legs straight. Slowly bend forward. Place the hands behind the knees. Pull the head down toward the knees. Hold for 5 counts. Relax. Repeat 3 times.

Perfection pull

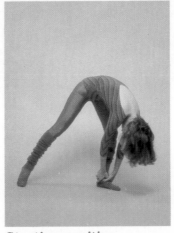

Starting position

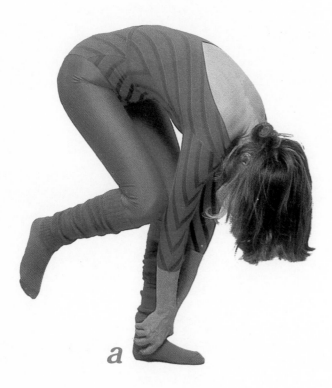

a

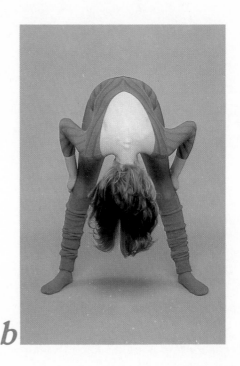

b

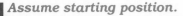
Assume starting position.

a Keep the left knee bent, hands on the ankle. Lift the right foot off the floor and bring the knee up toward the chest. Return to starting position. Repeat 15 times with each leg.

b Stand with feet wide apart, legs straight. Slowly bend forward. Place the hands behind the knees. Pull the head down toward the knees. Hold for 5 counts. Relax. Repeat 3 times.

Hip, hip away

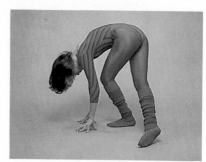

Starting position

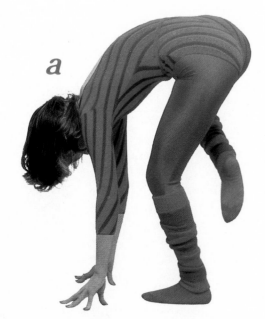

a

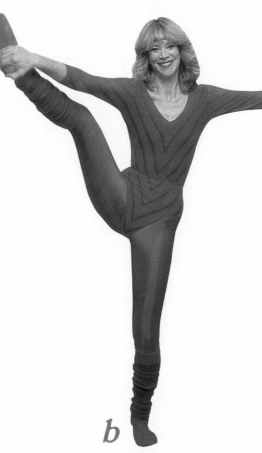

b

Assume starting position.

a Lift the right foot off the floor, bringing the knee up toward the chest. Return to starting position. Repeat 10 times with each leg.

b Stand, weight on left leg. Lift the right leg, placing right hand on the inside of the foot. Extend the leg up to the side. Straighten the leg as much as possible. Hold for 3 counts. Do once with each leg.

The thigh shaper

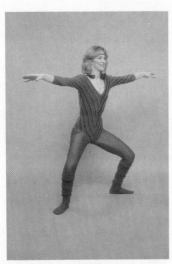

Starting position

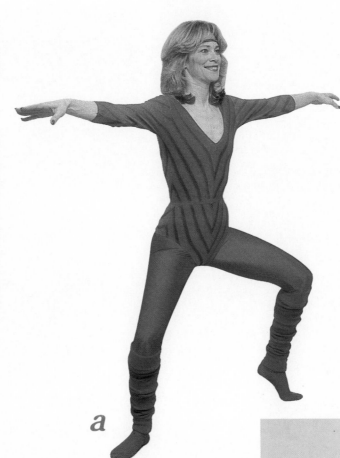

a

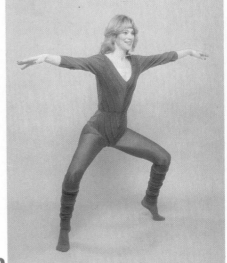

b

Assume starting position.

a Lift the left heel, keeping toes on the floor. Return heel to floor. Repeat with right heel. Alternate lifting left heel then right heel 20 times.

b Rest for 10 counts. Now lift and lower both heels at the same time. Repeat 20 times.

Lift and circle

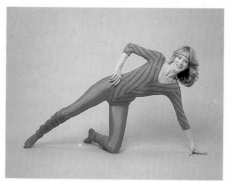

Starting position

Assume starting position.

a Raise the right leg up to the side as high as possible.

b Lower right leg so it is parallel to the floor. Then move the leg in a large circle to the side. Return to starting position. Repeat (lifting up, then circling) 5 times with the right leg, 5 times with the left leg. Repeat the sequence 3 times.

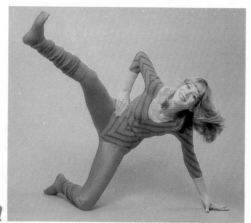

a

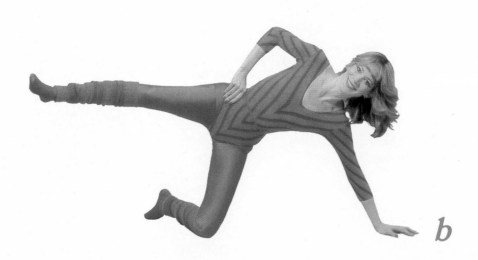

b

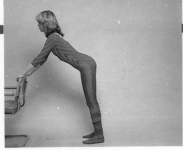

Starting position

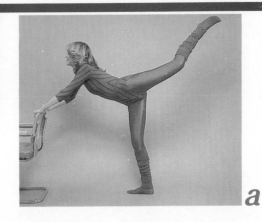

a

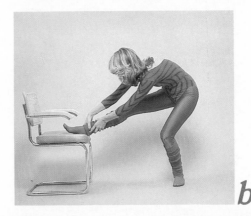

b

Cool down
Kick out

> *Assume starting position.*
>
> *a* Holding the back of a chair, lift the left knee up toward the chest. Then extend the left leg out in back. Repeat, bringing knee to chest and extending leg, 10 times with each leg.
>
> *b* Place right foot on the seat of the chair. Bend the left knee. Slowly reach hands to right ankle. Hold 5 counts. Do once with each leg.

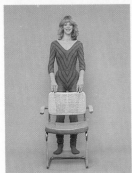

Starting position

Cool down
The pendulum

> *Assume starting position.*
>
> *a* Keep hands on the back of a chair. Swing the right leg across the body to the left side. Then swing the leg across to the right side. Raise the leg as high as possible. Swing each leg side to side 15 times. Be careful not to hit the toes on the chair as you swing across.
>
> *b* Place the right foot on the seat of the chair. Keep both legs straight. Slowly reach hands to the right ankle. Hold for 5 counts. Do once with each leg.

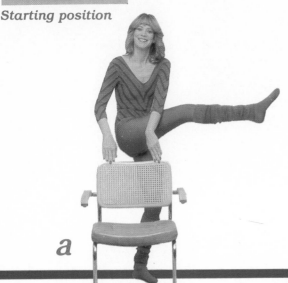

a

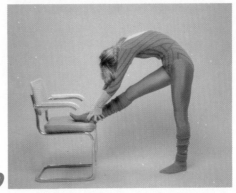

b

DAY 5

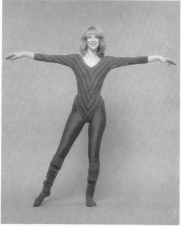

Starting position

Warm up
Chorus line I

Assume starting position.

a Hop on the left foot, touching the right foot to the floor behind the left foot. At the same time, cross the arms in front of the chest. Hop on the left foot again, returning the right foot and the arms to starting position. Repeat 20 times with each foot.

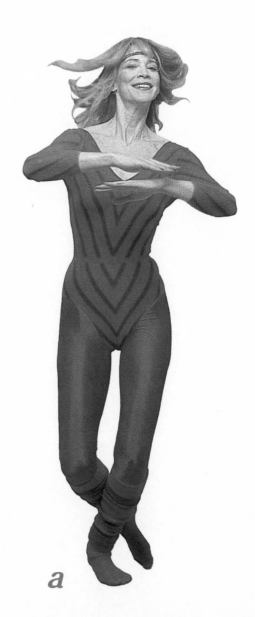

a

Warm up
Chorus line II

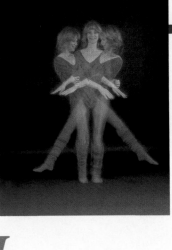

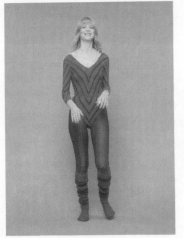

Starting position

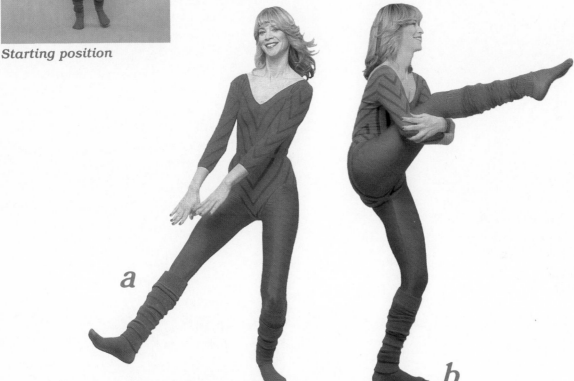

a

b

Assume starting position.

a Hop on the left foot, kicking the right foot out to the side, swinging the arms down toward the right leg. Jump, feet together. Then hop on the right foot, kicking the left foot out to the side, swinging arms down toward the left leg. Return to jump in the center. Repeat 20 times.

b Bring the right knee up to the chest, arms encircling the leg, hands holding the elbows. Slowly raise the leg as high as possible. Hold 5 counts. Do once with each leg.

The donkey

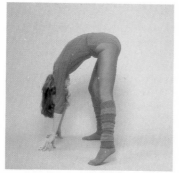

Starting position

Assume starting position.

a Keep fingertips on the floor. Bend the left knee in toward the chest.

b Then extend the leg directly to the side. Try to extend the leg at the height of the hip.

c Bend the knee in to the chest again. Extend the leg straight back. Repeat (knee in, leg to side, knee in, leg back) 10 times with each leg. Gradually work up to 20 times with each leg.

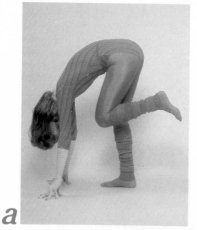

a

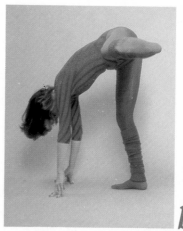

b

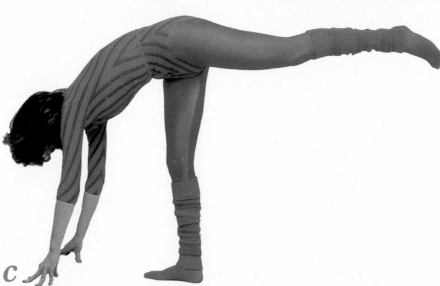

c

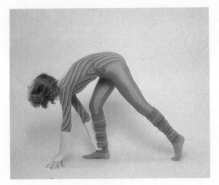

Starting position

The pivot

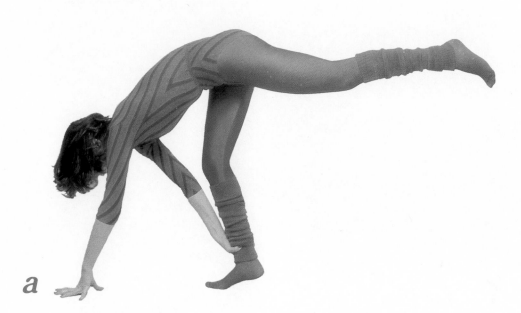

a

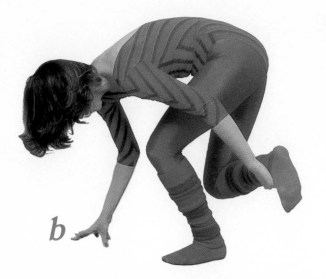

b

Assume starting position.

a Keep the left hand on the floor, right hand on the right ankle. Raise the left leg up in back and hold in that position. Lift the right heel and turn it to the left and the right 10 times, pivoting on the toes. Reverse leg positions and pivot 10 times on the left foot. Gradually work up to 20 times with each foot.

b Stand. Rest for 10 counts. Then bend the left knee. Place the right hand on the floor. Grasp the right ankle with the left hand. Slowly lower the right knee as close to the floor as possible. Then try to straighten the left leg. Repeat 5 times with each leg.

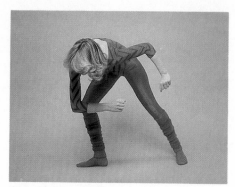

Starting position

Assume starting position.

a Lean torso over bent right knee. Turn both heels side to side, pivoting on the balls of the feet. At the same time, swing the arms side to side at knee level. Repeat for 5 counts.

b Bend lower and continue pivoting heels, swinging the arms at the ankle level, for 5 counts. Repeat (5 counts at knee level, 5 counts at ankle level) 10 times over the right knee, 10 times over the left knee.

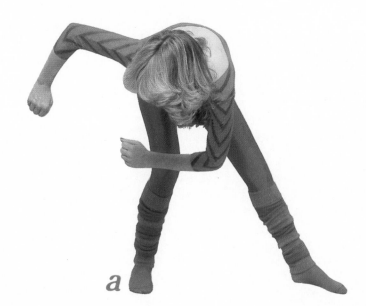

a

Double *pivot*

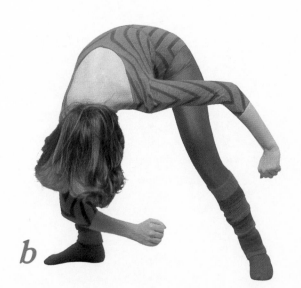

b

The arch

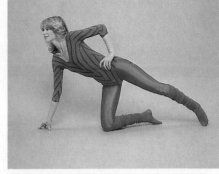

Starting position

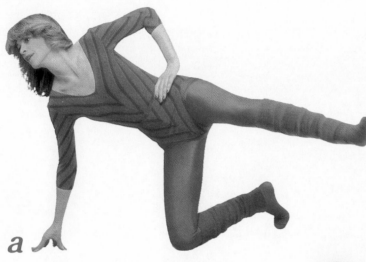

a

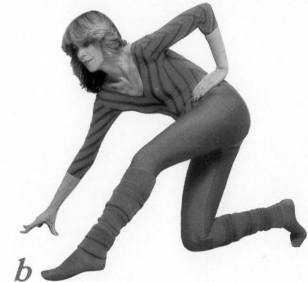

b

Assume starting position.

a Swing the left leg forward and up to the side as high as possible.

b Continue bringing the leg forward to touch the floor in front. Do this in one continuous movement, forming an imaginary arch with the leg. Then swing the leg in an arch back to the starting position. Swing forward and back 10 times with each leg.

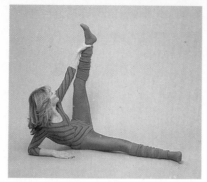

Starting position

Assume starting position.

a Keep the left hand on the left ankle. Lift the right leg up from the side to meet the left leg.

b Lower the right leg directly forward to the floor. Lift right leg straight up again. Then return the leg to the floor directly to the side. Repeat (up, forward, up, side) 10 times with each leg.

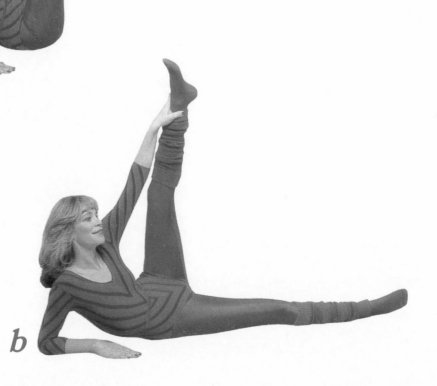

a

b

Daddy long legs

46

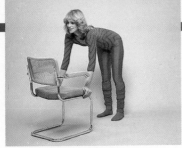

Starting position

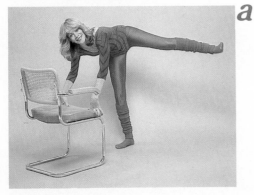

a

Cool down
Chair champs I

a Keep hands on the seat of the chair. Lift the left leg to hip height. Swing the leg forward to the side, then back. Repeat 15 times with each leg.

b Place the right foot on the seat of the chair. Turn the toes out to the side, so that the outer edge of the foot rests on the chair. Bend the left knee. Slowly reach hands to the right ankle. Hold for 5 counts. Do once with each leg.

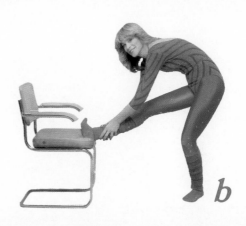

b

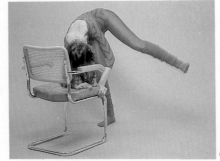

Starting position

Cool down
Chair champs II

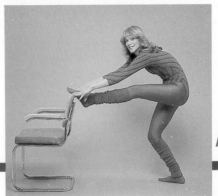

a

Assume starting position.

a Keep the right forearm on the seat of the chair, left hand gripping the chair. Move the left leg in large circles to the side 15 times. Then place the left forearm on the chair and circle the right leg 15 times.

b Place the left foot on top of the back of the chair. Bend the right knee to grasp the back of the chair. Slowly bend the right knee further down, then up, 5 times. Reverse leg positions and bounce 5 times with the left knee.

b

Warm up
The Charleston I

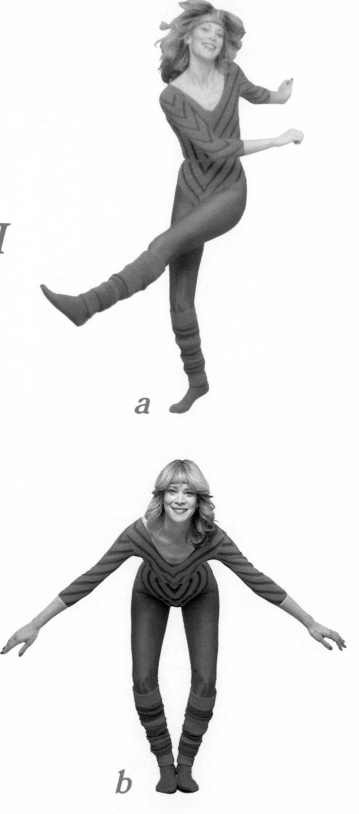
a

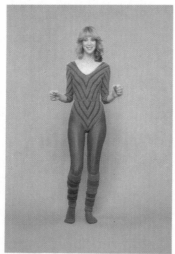

Starting position

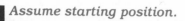
b

Assume starting position.

a Hop on the right foot, kicking the left leg across to the right. At the same time, swing the arms to the left. Jump, feet together. Then hop on the left foot, kicking the right leg across to the left, swinging the arms to the right. Return to jump in center. Repeat 10 times.

b Place feet together, knees bent. Open the knees, extending arms out to the sides. Then close the knees, crossing the arms above the knees. Repeat 5 times.

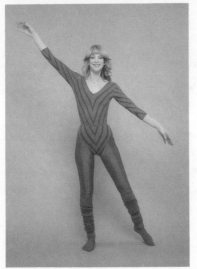

Starting position

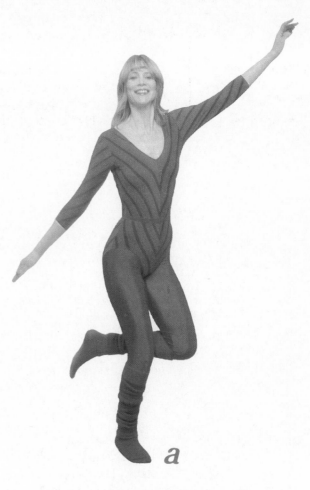

a

Warm up
The Charleston II

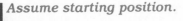

Assume starting position.

a Hop on the right foot, kicking the left foot up behind the right. Touch the foot with the right hand. Jump, feet together. Then hop on the left foot, kicking the right foot up behind the left. Touch the right foot with the left hand. Return to jump in the center. Repeat 10 times.

b Place the hands on the hips. Raise the shoulders. Shake the right leg for 5 counts. Then shake the left leg for 5 counts.

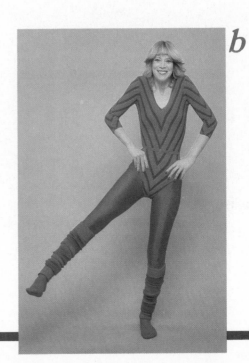

b

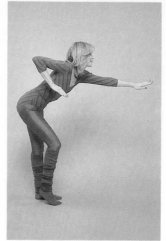

Starting position

Reach out

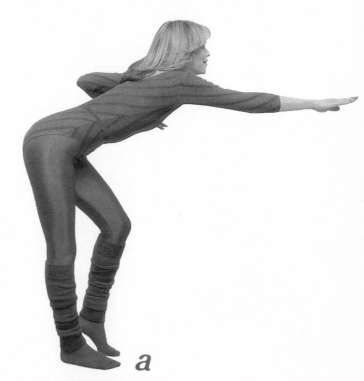

Assume starting position.

a Press the right heel down, straightening the right leg. Reach the right arm straight forward. At the same time, bend the left knee, lift the left heel, and pull the left elbow back. Alternately lift heels, switching arm positions, 30 times. (If your back is weak, do not lean forward. Do the exercise upright.)

b Kneel, hands on the floor, head down. Round the back by pulling up on the abdominal muscles. Hold for 5 counts. Then slowly flatten the back. Hold for 5 counts. Round and flatten the back 3 times.

a

b

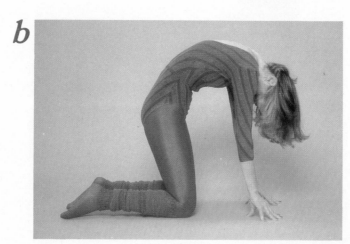

Circle & kick magic

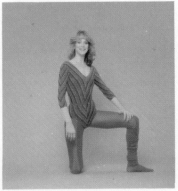

Starting position

Assume starting position.

a Bending from the waist, swing the right arm forward and up.

b Continue circling the arm up overhead and back.

c On the back swing, lean back to place the right hand on the floor. Lift the left leg as high as possible, touching the ankle with the left hand. Return to starting position. Repeat 15 times with each leg.

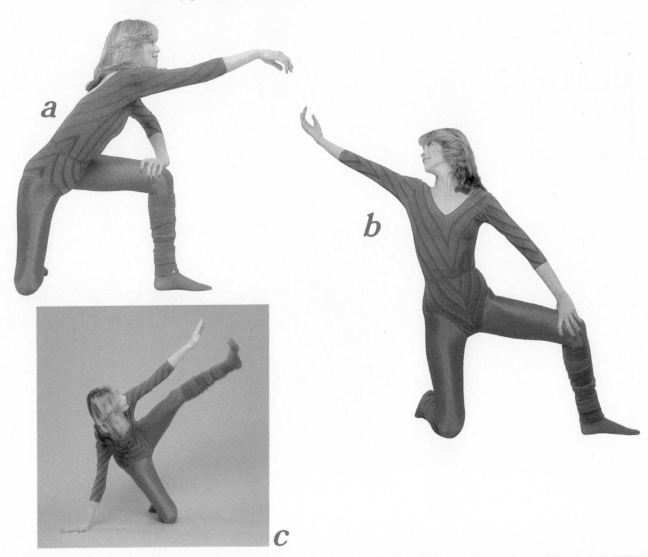

a

b

c

Hamstring stretch

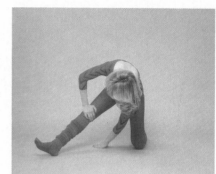

Starting position

Assume starting position.

a Keep left hand on the floor under the right knee, right toes up, right hand on the knee to support the back. Bend the left elbow down to the floor. Then straighten the elbow. Repeat 10 times. Reverse arm and leg positions and repeat with the right elbow 10 times.

b In the starting position, place the right foot flat on the floor. Place the left hand on the floor behind the right heel. Bend the left elbow to the floor and straighten 10 times. Reverse arm and leg positions and repeat with the right elbow 10 times.

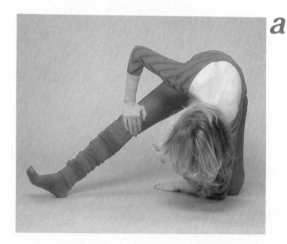

a

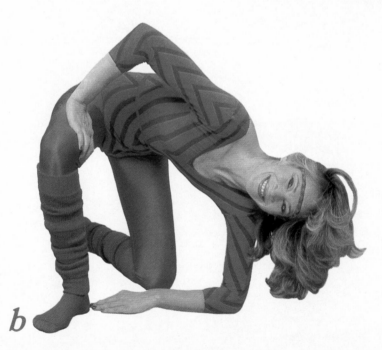

b

$\mathcal{H}$ip lifter

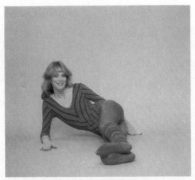

Starting position

Assume starting position.

a Raise both legs straight up from the side.

b Then lower legs forward to the floor. Lift legs up again. Then return to the floor at the side. Repeat 5 times to the right side, 5 times to the left side. Work up to 10 times each side.

c Sit, right leg straight forward on the floor. Cross the left foot to the floor outside the right knee. Grasp the left ankle with both hands. Pull the head down toward the ankle. Hold for 5 counts. Do once with each foot.

a

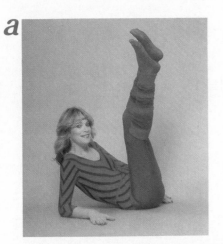

b

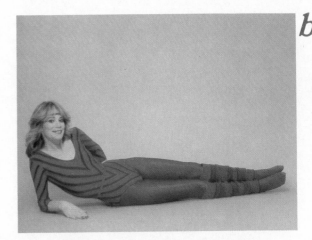

c

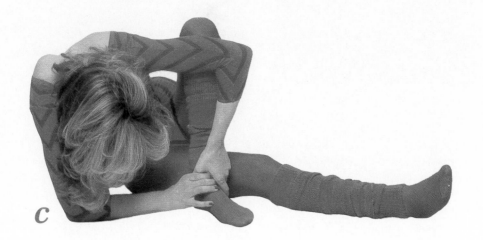

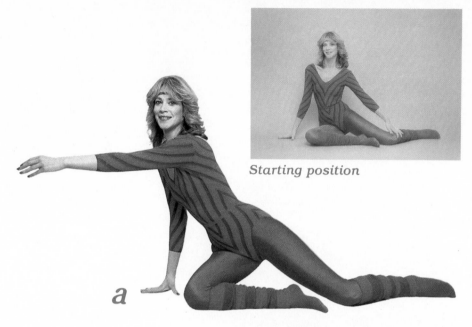

Starting position

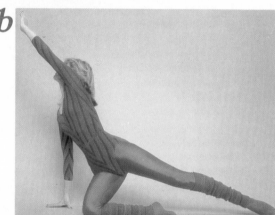

a

S*weep up*

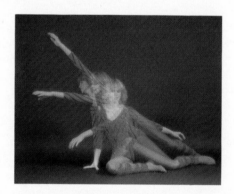

Assume starting position.

a Lift the hips off the floor, shifting the weight to the right hand and knee. Swing the left arm forward at the same time.

b Continue the motion, lifting hips higher, extending the left leg straight back, swinging the left arm up. Then swing back down to the starting position. Repeat 10 times to each side.

b

Cool down
The table

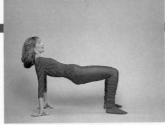

Starting position

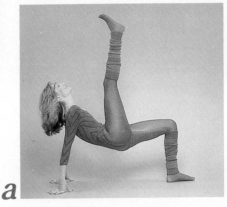

a

Assume starting position.

a Lift the right leg and bend the knee in toward the chest. Then kick the leg straight up.

b Bend the knee in toward the chest again. Then kick the leg straight forward. Repeat (knee in, kick up, knee in, kick forward) 15 times with each leg.

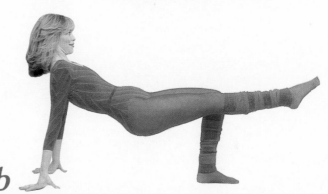

b

Cool down
Jumping bean

Assume starting position.

a Jump up and down, keeping knees slightly bent. Land lightly on the feet. Jump 20 times. Work up to 30 times.

b Place the right leg forward, knee bent, in a lunge position. Extend the left leg back. Turn the right foot to the side. Clasp the right ankle with both hands. Slowly straighten the right leg. Bend and straighten the leg 5 times. Reverse leg positions and repeat 5 times with the left leg.

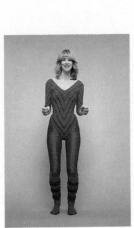

Starting position

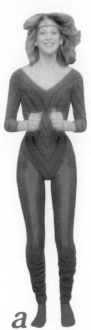

a

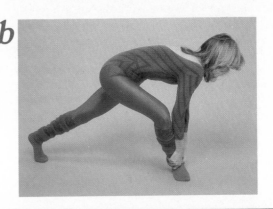

b

Warm up
The dancer

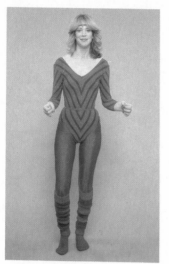

Starting position

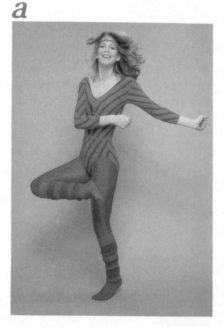

a

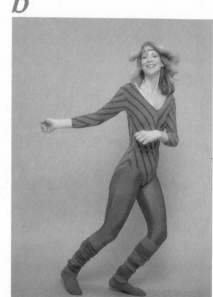

b

Assume starting position.

a Hop on the left foot, lifting the right knee up to the side, turning torso to the right. At the same time, swing both arms to the left.

b Hop on the left foot again, returning the right foot to the floor. At the same time, turn torso to the left, swinging arms to the right. Repeat 10 times with each leg.

c Bend the right knee up toward the chest. Hold the bottom of the foot with both hands. Slowly straighten the leg as much as possible. Hold for 5 counts. Lower foot to the floor. Do once with each leg.

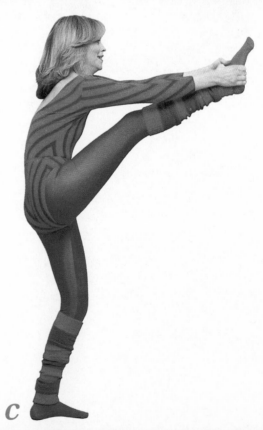

c

Starting position

Warm up
Keep dancing

Assume starting position.

a Step to the right and leap on the right foot, landing with right knee bent. On the leap, swing the arms up to the right and extend the left leg up to the side. Then step to the left and leap on the left foot, swinging arms up to the left, right leg up to the side. Leap right then left 10 times.

b Stand with the feet together. Bend the knees. Place the hands on the floor outside the feet, fingers turned back.

c Very slowly try to straighten the legs, keeping the hands flat on the floor. Hold for 5 counts. Relax. Then slowly uncurl the back and return to an upright position. (If you have a weak back, do not straighten the knees completely. Straighten only until you feel a pull in the back of the legs.)

a

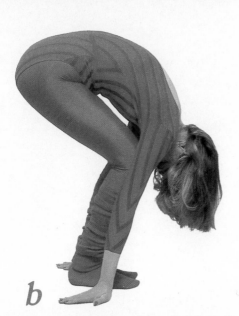

b

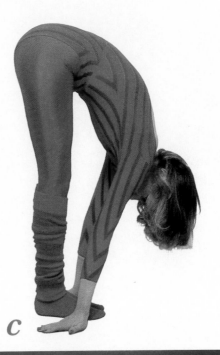

c

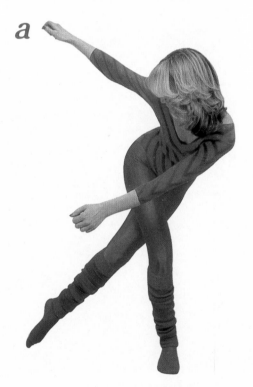

Starting position

Figure shaper I

Assume starting position.

a Bending the right knee slightly, cross the left leg behind the right, touching foot to the floor. At the same time, swing the arms down and across to the right. Return to starting position. Repeat 10 times with each leg.

b Cross the left leg behind the right. Place both hands on the right knee. Bend and straighten the right leg 5 times. Then reverse leg positions and repeat 5 times with the left leg.

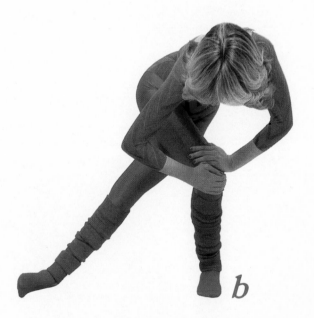

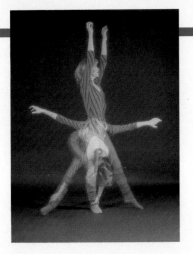

Assume starting position.

a Bending the right knee slightly, cross the left leg behind the right, touching the foot to the floor. At the same time, swing the hands down to touch the ankles. Return to starting position. Repeat 10 times with each leg.

b Cross the left leg behind the right. Hold the ankles. Slowly try to straighten both legs in a long stretch. Hold for 5 counts. Then reverse leg positions and repeat the stretch. Do once with each leg.

*F*igure *s*haper II

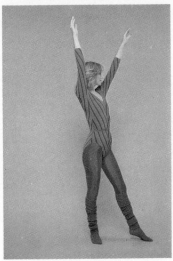

Starting position

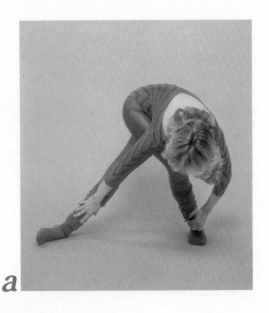

a

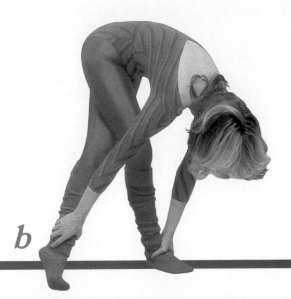

b

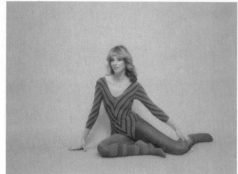
Starting position

*U*p, up, and away

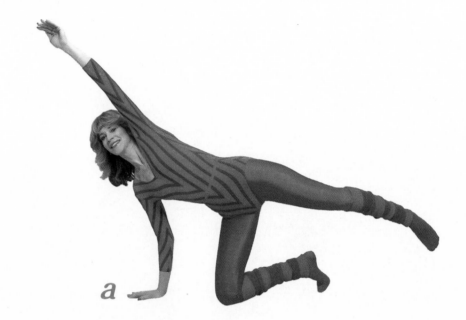

a

b

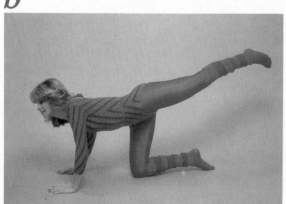

Assume starting position.

a Shifting the weight to the right hand and knee, lift the torso. Swing the left arm forward and up, lifting the left leg straight back.

b Then place both hands on the floor, bending the elbows. Lift the left leg up in back as high as possible. Return to starting position. Repeat 10 times with each leg. Try to flow in this exercise, going from the starting position to the leg lift in one smooth motion.

Lift-off

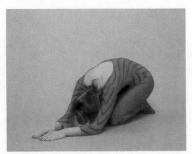

Starting position

Assume starting position.

a Lift the torso. With weight on the right hand and knee, extend the left arm forward, the left leg back. Return to starting position. Repeat 10 times with the left arm and leg, 10 times with the right arm and leg.

b Kneel with the right hand on the floor. Grasp the left knee with the left hand. Pull the knee up toward the chest, pressing the head down toward the knee. Hold for 5 counts. Do once with each leg.

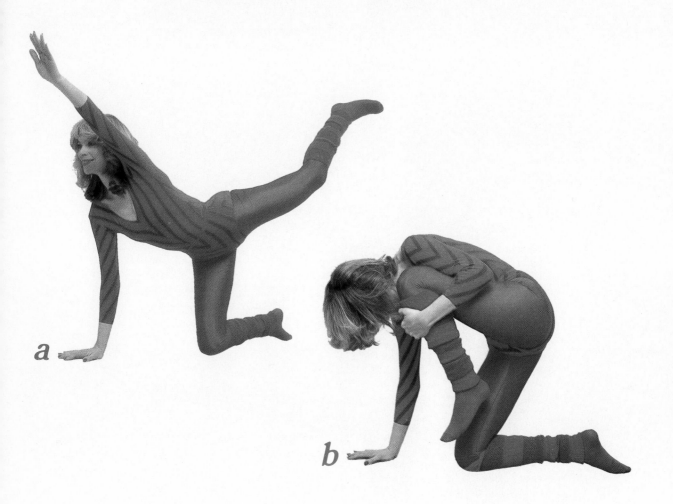

a

b

Circle sweep

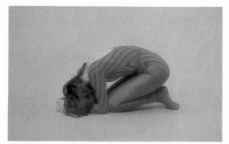

Starting position

Assume starting position.

a With weight on the right hand and knee, lift the torso. Bring the left knee and left arm forward.

b Extend the leg up to the side. Swing the arm to the side to follow the motion of the leg.

c Swing the leg and arm straight back. Return to starting position. Repeat 10 times with each leg. Try to do this exercise in one smooth motion. Form an imaginary circle as the arm and leg move forward, side, back, and down to the starting position.

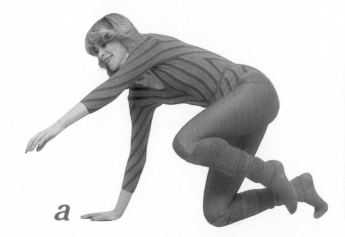

a

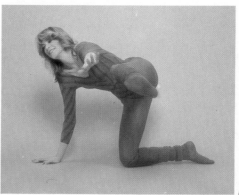

b

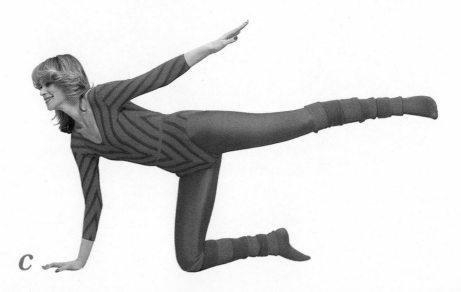

c

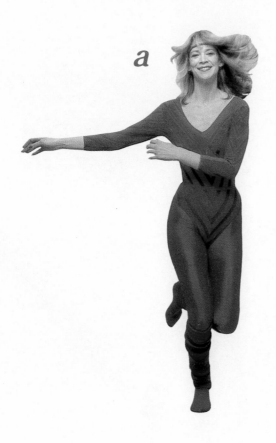

Starting position

Cool down
Ragtime reviver

Assume starting position.

a Hop on the right foot, bending the left knee to cross the left leg up behind the right. At the same time, swing arms to the right. Then jump, feet together.

b Hop on the left foot, bending the right knee to cross the right leg up behind the left. Swing arms to the left. Return to jump in the center. Kick up left leg then right leg 30 times.

a

b

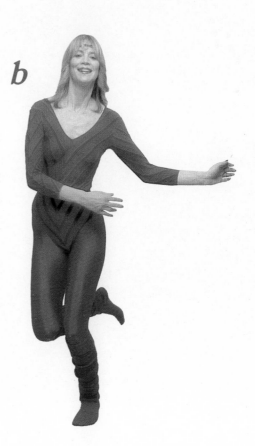

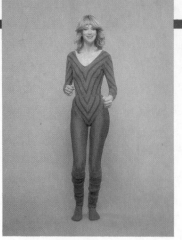

Starting position

Assume starting position.

a Lift knees in an easy run-in-place for 30 counts. Gradually increase the counts as you build up strength.

b Stand with the feet wide apart. Extend the right arm up. Grasp the elbow with the left hand. Pull the right arm across to the left. Stretch for 5 counts. Do once with each arm.

a

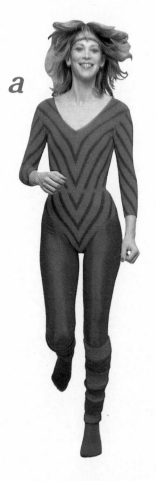

Cool down
Energy booster

b

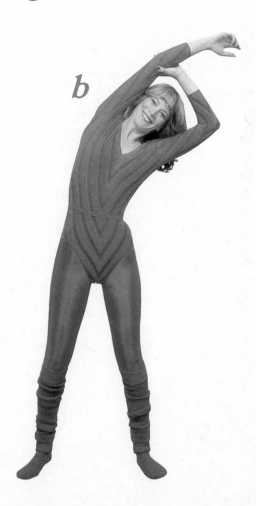